# Designing and Conducting Clinical Trials – An overview

## Preface

Clinical trials can be defined as an experiment which is conducted in a controlled environment to test the efficacy of drugs, procedures, methodology before bringing into the public domain. The clinical trials started in $2^{nd}$ century BC by Daniel & King Nebuchadnezzar. Formal recorded therapeutic clinical trial was started way back in 1537 AD by a Surgeon. Current clinical trials include clear guidelines, adhering to regulatory requirements, getting consent from the patients, ensuring safety of the patients, adopting ethical practices, close monitoring of the trials and using advanced statistical tools to analyze and report the findings.

Advancement in technology such as cloud computing, big data analytics, machine learning algorithms, data base management and advanced statistical software helped to transform the different stages of clinical trials - the data collection, data storage, data monitoring, data management and data analysis.

This book provides an overview of clinical trials, different phases & types of clinical trial, randomization, blinding, allocation, ethical issues, protocol, data collection forms, data management, data analysis and reporting of the clinical trial.

It is recommended to refer author's book on Application of Statistical Tools in Biomedical Domain: An Overview with Help of Software (**https://www.amazon.com/dp/1986988554**) and Essentials of Bio-Statistics: An overview with the help of Software if you need to familiarize yourself with the basic statistical knowledge.

**Editor,** International Journal of Statistics and Medical Informatics

Chapter 1 - Clinical Trial History.............................................. 3

Chapter 2 – Phases of Clinical Trials ......................................... 7

Chapter 3 – Types of Clinical Trials........................................... 10

Chapter 4 – Clinical Trial Protocol ........................................... 12

Chapter 5 – Clinical Trials Designs........................................... 14

Chapter 6 – Hypothesis and Sample size determination .......... 21

Chapter 7 – Patient allocation and blinding............................. 34

Chapter 8 – Data collection and Data monitoring during the clinical trial ........................................................................... 44

Chapter 9 – Statistical Analysis in clinical trial ......................... 48

Chapter 10 – Reporting in clinical trial .................................... 52

# Chapter 1 - Clinical Trial History

This chapter provides the history and progress made in the clinical trials, its process, regulatory and ethical requirements. The following table provides the time line of the clinical trials conducted in the past

### Table 1.1 – History of the clinical trials

| S.no | Name of the investigator | Year | Trial description | Characteristics |
|------|---------------------------|------|-------------------|-----------------|
| 1 | Daniel and King Nebuchadnezzar | 2nd Century BC | Diet comparison | First clinical trial |
| 2 | Ambroise Paré | 1537 | Therapy for battlefield wounds | First formal recorded therapeutic trial |
| 3 | Dr. James Lind | 1747 | Treatment for Scurvy | A Comparative study |
| 4 | Robert Robertson | 1776 | Bark study | A Comparative study |
| 5 | Austin Flint | 1863 | Treatment for rheumatic fever | Introduction of Placebo |
| 6 | Medical Research Council | 1934-44 | Treatment for common cold - Patulin | Double blind trail |
| 7 | Dr. Amberson | 1924 | Treatment of pulmonary tuberculosis | Randomization in clinical trail |

| S. no | Name of the investigator | Year | Trial description | Characteristics |
|---|---|---|---|---|
| 8 | Austin Bradford Hill and Philip Hart – Medical research council | 1976 | tests of streptomycin for the treatment of tuberculosis | Randomization in clinical trail |

**Other historical highlights of clinical trials and other studies**

- During the year 1854, John Snow the first epidemiologist found that Cholera was a water-borne disease (epidemiological study).
- During the year 1855, Florence Nightingale, a pioneer of nursing and a reformer of hospital sanitation used statistical analysis tools for collecting, recording and displaying the clinical data and showed evidence of improvement in the patient conditions.
- During the year 1906, United States of America created the Food and Drug Act and established Food and Drug Administration (FDA) Authority.
- During the year 1938, new upgraded FDA law which came into effect subjected new drugs to pre-market safety evaluation.
- During the year 1947, Nuremberg Code (International Code of Medical Ethics) was introduced to protect the human participation in the clinical trials.
- During the year 1962, FDA upgraded the act with use of scientific testing and ensuring evidence of drug's efficacy.

- During the year 1964, World Medical Association (WMA) came with the Declaration of Helsinki which focused on voluntary involvement and informed consent in the human subject research.
- During the year 1948, Framingham Heart Study (FHS) was started to identify common factors that contributed to cardiovascular disease (epidemiological study).
- During the year 1974, FDA created Bureau of Medical Devices and Diagnostic Products.
- During the year 1990, International Council for Harmonization (ICH) was established and developed harmonized guidelines for global pharmaceutical developments (Guidelines for Good Clinical Practice (GCP)).
- During the year 1996, United States of America introduced Health Insurance Portability and Accountability Act (HIPAA) .
- During the year 2000, ClinicalTrials.Gov website was launched by National Library of Medicine (NLM).
- During the year 2008, World Medical Association revised the Declaration of Helsinki with prospective registration and the public disclosure of study results to include ethical obligations.
- During the year 2012, FDA act was amended with Safety and innovation act which enables FDA to collect fees from the healthcare industry to fund the breakthrough therapy and innovative drugs.
- During the year 2019, FDA is considering a regulatory framework for Artificial Intelligence and Machine Learning technologies in health care (Software as a Medical Device)

**Reference**

1. Bhatt, A. (2010). Evolution of clinical research: a history before and beyond James Lind. Perspectives in clinical research, 1(1), 6.
2. Greenfield, M. L. (2013). Of Plagues, Blights, and Bloodletting: Historical Highlights of the Randomized Controlled Trial.
3. Junod, S. W. (2014). FDA and clinical drug trials: a short history. US Food and Drug Administration.
4. Nellhaus, E. M., & Davies, T. H. (2017). Evolution of Clinical Trials throughout History. Marshall Journal of Medicine, 3(1), 41.
5. Paneth, N. (2004). Assessing the contributions of John Snow to epidemiology: 150 years after removal of the broad street pump handle. Epidemiology, 15(5), 514-516.
6. https://www.fda.gov/
7. https://www.clinicaltrials.gov/
8. https://www.wma.net/
9. https://www.fda.gov/MedicalDevices/DigitalHealth/SoftwareasaMedicalDevice/ucm634612.htm
10. https://history.nih.gov/research/downloads/nuremberg.pdf
11. https://www.framinghamheartstudy.org/
12. https://www.ich.org/about/history.html
13. https://www.ich.org/fileadmin/Public_Web_Site/ICH_Products/Guidelines/Efficacy/E6/E6_R1_Guideline.pdf
14. https://www.fda.gov/downloads/MedicalDevices/DigitalHealth/SoftwareasaMedicalDevice/UCM635052.pdf
15. https://www.hhs.gov/hipaa/index.html

# Chapter 2 – Phases of Clinical Trials

Clinical trials are conducted in different phases based on experimental subject, nature and objective of the study. The table explains different phases of clinical trials and its significance.

**Table 2.1 – Phases of clinical trials**

| Phases | Type | Objective | Experimental subjects |
|---|---|---|---|
| **Phase-0 or preclinical trail phase** | Initial safety trial | 1.  To test the safety of the drug | 1.  Usually animals |
| **Phase-1** | safety trial | 1.  To test the pharmacodynamics /Pharmacokinetics characteristics<br>2.  To Find out the dose range | 1.  Severely ill patients or without disease (Volunteers)<br>2.  Number of patients is less |
| **Phase-II** | Efficacy and safety trial | 1.  To find out dose response<br>2.  To find out frequency of dosage<br>3.  To find out the efficacy | 1.  Normal Patients with disease condition<br>2.  Larger than Phase-1 |

| Phases | Type | Objective | Experimental subjects |
|---|---|---|---|
| **Phase III** | Efficacy and safety trial before regulatory approval | 1. Find out more information on efficacy and safety of the drugs 2. To Compare efficacy of old/placebo drug with new drug | 1. Target patient population with disease condition 2. Require more number of patients than phase-II 3. Patients with different characteristics 4. Randomized, controlled and blinded |
| **Phase IV** | Post marketing of the drugs | 1. To assess Adverse events 2. To test New category of patients 3. To find More information on efficacy and safety | 1. To assess the long term benefit 2. Larger Patient population 3. To assess Cost benefit |

**References**

1. Mahan, V. L. (2014). Clinical trial phases. International Journal of Clinical Medicine, 5(21), 1374.

2. Sedgwick, P. (2014). What are the four phases of clinical research trials?. BMJ, 348, g3727.

3. **https://www.cancerresearchuk.org/about-cancer/find-a-clinical-trial/what-clinical-trials-are/phases-of-clinical-trials**

4. Ivy, S. P., Siu, L. L., Garrett-Mayer, E., & Rubinstein, L. (2010). Approaches to phase 1 clinical trial design focused on safety, efficiency, and selected patient populations: a report from the clinical trial design task force of the national cancer institute investigational drug steering committee. Clinical Cancer Research, 16(6), 1726-1736.

5. Seymour, L., Ivy, S. P., Sargent, D., Spriggs, D., Baker, L., Rubinstein, L., ... & Groshen, S. (2010). The design of phase II clinical trials testing cancer therapeutics: consensus recommendations from the clinical trial design task force of the national cancer institute investigational drug steering committee. Clinical Cancer Research, 16(6), 1764-1769.

6. Thall, P. F. (2008). A review of phase 2–3 clinical trial designs. Lifetime data analysis, 14(1), 37-53.

7. Zhang, X., Zhang, Y., Ye, X., Guo, X., Zhang, T., & He, J. (2016). Overview of phase IV clinical trials for postmarket drug safety surveillance: a status report from the ClinicalTrials. gov registry. BMJ open, 6(11), e010643.

8. Bahadur, N. (2008). Overview of drug development. Emerging Growth Markets. Bangkok, 17.

# Chapter 3 – Types of Clinical Trials

There are different types clinical trials such as treatment, diagnostic, vaccine or preventive, behavioral, quality of life trials conducted based on the nature of the problem.

### Treatment trials
Treatment trials are conduced to assess the efficacy of new drugs or treatments or therapies. Treatment trials are conducted in different phases (pre-clinical to Phase IV). These trials involve compassion between drugs and participants are allocated to group in random manner. Testing for equality, superiority, non-inferiority and equivalence treatment trails are conducted to assess the equality or superiority or equivalence or non-inferiority among the treatment methodologies or drugs.

### Diagnostic trials
Diagnostic trails are conducted to assess whether new test or diagnosis help to detect or screen the disease at the early stage. The study population in these trials will be general population or people with high risk of developing disease condition.

### Vaccine or preventive trials
Vaccine or preventive trials are conducted to assess risk of disease and possibility of reducing the risks. The study participants in these trials will be from the high risk group.

### Behavioral trials

Behavioral trials are conducted to assess the impact of behavioral intervention on the disease condition.

### Quality of life trials

These trials are conducted to assess whether quality of life of the patients is improved or not, side effects are reduced or not.

### Single or multi center trials

There are two different types of clinical trials are conducted based on the location: single center and multi center trials.

Single center trials are conducted at one single entity like hospital, clinical research center with less number of patients wherein the multi-center trials involve number of trials centers spread of over cities or countries.

Multi central trials involve large number of patients and the findings of the trials are mostly generalizable to larger population than the single center trial.

Single center trials are less complex and less expensive than the multi-center trials.

### References

1.      https://www.australianclinicaltrials.gov.au/types-clinical-trials
2.      https://www.cancer.gov/about-cancer/treatment/clinical-trials/what-are-trials/types

# Chapter 4 – Clinical Trial Protocol

Clinical trial protocol contains all the information about a clinical trial. A good clinical trial protocol usually follows guidelines set by International Conference on Harmonization (ICH).

Normally the clinical trial protocols contain the following information (not limited to).

1. Protocol number, title, date, sponsor details, trial center details
2. Trial objectives and Rationale
3. Background information
4. Risk and benefits
5. Treatment details
6. Clinical trial designs
7. Randomization procedures
8. Inclusion and exclusion criteria
9. Sample size
10. Evaluation of treatment efficacy and safety
11. Trial Stopping Rule
12. Adverse event details
13. Participants withdrawal information
14. Ethical guidelines
15. Data collection and monitoring procedures
16. Statistical analysis
17. Clinical trial timelines
18. Financial or funding information
19. Publication details
20. References

**References**
1. https://www.ich.org/products/guidelines
2. Bhuiyan, P. S., & Rege, N. N. (2001). ICH Harmonised Tripartite Guideline: guideline for good clinical practice.
3. Lewis, J. A. (1999). Statistical principles for clinical trials (ICH E9): an introductory note on an international guideline. Statistics in medicine, 18(15), 1903-1942.
4. Chan, A. W., Tetzlaff, J. M., Altman, D. G., Laupacis, A., Gøtzsche, P. C., Krleža-Jerić, K., ... & Doré, C. J. (2013). SPIRIT 2013 statement: defining standard protocol items for clinical trials. Annals of internal medicine, 158(3), 200-207.
5. Vijayananthan, A., & Nawawi, O. (2008). The importance of Good Clinical Practice guidelines and its role in clinical trials. Biomedical imaging and intervention journal, 4(1).
6. Gamble, C., Krishan, A., Stocken, D., Lewis, S., Juszczak, E., Doré, C., ... & Berlin, J. (2017). Guidelines for the content of statistical analysis plans in clinical trials. Jama, 318(23), 2337-2343.
7. Brody, T. (2016). Clinical trials: study design, endpoints and biomarkers, drug safety, and FDA and ICH guidelines. Academic press.
8. Verma, K. (2013). Base of a research: good clinical practice in clinical trials. J Clin Trials, 3(1), 100-28.
9. Tetzlaff, J. M., Chan, A. W., Kitchen, J., Sampson, M., Tricco, A. C., & Moher, D. (2012). Guidelines for randomized clinical trial protocol content: a systematic review. Systematic reviews, 1(1), 43.

# Chapter 5 – Clinical Trials Designs

Clinical trials involve different types of trial designs such as Randomized Clinical Trials (RCTs), cross over design, factorial design, cluster design, historical controls. The choice of design depends on the objective of the study, study population characteristics and Impact on the outcome of the study.

**Randomized Clinical Trial (RCT) design**
Randomized Clinical Trial design is the widely used design in the clinical trials. The patients are randomly allocated to the treatment group and control group. The control group will be usually a standard treatment (drug) group or placebo or no treatment at all.  RCT design allocates patient to only one group and receive only one treatment or drug.
*Advantages of RCTs*
1. It avoids bias in allocation
2. The results of the clinical trial will be valid and reduces allocation bias

*Disadvantages of RCT*
3. Generalizability of the results might be difficult for the whole patient population
4. Participants may refuse to be in one of the group would want to switch over to the other group after randomization.

**Factorial designs**

Factorial designs involve assessing of two or more factors (treatments or drugs) at the same clinical trial. The factorial design can be a complete (3x3) or incomplete design (2x3).

*Advantages*
1. Able to compare two treatments simultaneously
2. Reduces the cost of the trials

*Disadvantages*
3. Interaction between treatments or drugs will be a problem.
4. Participants might not be willing to take treatments or drugs combination at a time.
5. Finding the right dosage of drugs combination might be a problem.

**Cross over designs**

The cross over designs involves allocating of patients in both treatment and control groups at different period of time in a clinical trial.

*Advantages*
1. Removes the individual patient effect from the drug effect
2. More informative than the RCT

*Disadvantages*
1. Carry over effect between drugs and treatment may affect the outcome of the whole trial
2. Often difficult to determine the optimum switch over period for drugs.

## Cluster Randomized Clinical Trial Design

Cluster Randomized clinical trial design involves random allocation of the treatment or control group to group or cluster of patients not at the level of the individual patients. The group may include patients living in a city or community. The patients will have similar characteristics among them but vary with other group or cluster of patients.

*Advantages*
1. Feasible than RCTs - More easy to identify and recruit patients
2. Helpful in Public Health field related studies

*Disadvantages*
1. Require large sample size
2. Analysis and Interpretation of results will be difficult than RCTs

## Matched pair clinical trial design

In matched pair design, patients who are having similar characteristics are matched in pair and one of the patient from each pair is allocated to treatment and control group.

*Advantages*
1. Reduces the patient effect as patients in both control and treatment group are comparable

*Disadvantages*
1. Identifying variables for creating the matching pairs might be difficult

**Adaptive clinical trial design**

Adaptive clinical trial design uses the results of the clinical trial during the conduct of the trial and updates the parameters, direction and design of the trial. Interim analysis will be carried out to check the efficacy of the treatment.

*Advantages*

1. Flexible than fixed design
2. Saves time and cost
3. Requires less number of patients in the study
4. Ethically advantageous than fixed design as trials can be stopped if the treatment found to be non-effective at the early stage of the study

*Disadvantages*

1. The acceptance of adaptive designs are still in the early stages as it involves certain amount subjectivity in deciding the results of the trial in the early stage
2. Require more time to design the adaptive clinical trials
3. Interpretation and generalization of the results might be a problem as there is a possibility of getting different results after changing the trial parameters.

**Group Sequential clinical trial design**

In Group sequential clinical trial design, the patients are recruited sequentially in groups and interim and final analysis will be carried out at predefined intervals. If the results are positive then the trial will continue with more number of patients till final end point is reached or if the results are negative (example: life threatening effects) the trial will be stopped at that point itself. It is similar to adaptive clinical trial designs in terms of sample size requirement and interim analysis but the design parameters will not be changed it will remain fixed not like adaptive design wherein the design can be modified during the conduct of the trial..

*Advantages*
1. Requires less sample size
2. Saves time and cost
3. Ethically advantageous than fixed design as trials can be stopped if the treatment found to be non-effective at the early stage of the study

*Disadvantages*
1. Not flexible as adaptive clinical trial designs
2. Interpretation and generalization of the results might be a problem as there is a possibility of getting different results between the interim analysis and the final analysis.

# References

1. Stanley, K. (2007). Design of randomized controlled trials. Circulation, 115(9), 1164-1169.

2. Guerrera, F., Renaud, S., Tabbò, F., & Filosso, P. L. (2017). How to design a randomized clinical trial: tips and tricks for conduct a successful study in thoracic disease domain. Journal of thoracic disease, 9(8), 2692.

3. Green, S., Liu, P. Y., & O'sullivan, J. (2002). Factorial design considerations. Journal of Clinical Oncology, 20(16), 3424-3430.

4. Kendall, J. M. (2003). Designing a research project: randomised controlled trials and their principles. Emergency Medicine Journal, 20(2), 164-168.

5. Stampfer, M. J., Buring, J. E., Willett, W., Rosner, B., Eberlein, K., & Hennekens, C. H. (1985). The 2× 2 factorial design: Its application to a randomized trial of aspirin and US physicians. Statistics in medicine, 4(2), 111-116.

6. Jones, B., & Kenward, M. G. (2014). Design and analysis of cross-over trials. Chapman and Hall/CRC.

7. MERIT Study Investigators. (2005). Introduction of the medical emergency team (MET) system: a cluster-randomised controlled trial. The Lancet, 365(9477), 2091-2097.

8. Pallmann, P., Bedding, A. W., Choodari-Oskooei, B., Dimairo, M., Flight, L., Hampson, L. V., ... & Wason, J. M. (2018). Adaptive designs in clinical trials: why use them, and how to run and report them. BMC medicine, 16(1), 29.

9. GUIDANCE, D. (2018). Adaptive Designs for Clinical Trials of Drugs and Biologics. Center for Biologics Evaluation and Research (CBER).

10. Thorlund, K., Haggstrom, J., Park, J. J., & Mills, E. J. (2018). Key design considerations for adaptive clinical trials: a primer for clinicians. bmj, 360, k698.

11. Pocock, S. J. (1977). Group sequential methods in the design and analysis of clinical trials. Biometrika, 64(2), 191-199.

12. Kelly, P. J., Roshini Sooriyarachchi, M., Stallard, N., & Todd, S. (2005). A practical comparison of group-sequential and adaptive designs. Journal of Biopharmaceutical Statistics, 15(4), 719-738.

# Chapter 6 – Hypothesis and Sample size determination

Once the clinical trial objectives and design is finalized next step is to define the hypothesis, determine the sample size, randomization procedure, patient allocation to groups, types of blinding to be applied. We need to determine the inclusion and exclusion criteria, stop rules, interim analysis intervals based on the study design requirement.

**Formulation of Hypothesis**
Hypothesis statements include null and alternative hypothesis. The alternative hypothesis statement includes the research problem we are going to test and null hypothesis statement reflects the neutral state. For example, we would like to conduct a randomized clinical trial to test the efficacy of new cancer drug on lung cancer in comparison with the standard drug then the null and alternative hypothesis statement will be defined as follows:

**Null Hypothesis (H0):** There is no difference in the survival rate of the lung cancer patients with respect to standard and new drug groups

**Alternative Hypothesis (H1):** The survival rate of lung patient is more in new drug group than in the standard drug group.

If the difference between the survival rates is not statistically significant then the null hypothesis will be accepted and alternative hypothesis will be rejected. But there are situation wherein the null hypothesis may be wrongly rejected or accepted which might lead to the following errors

### Table 5.1 – Decision Matrix

| | Actual status of Null Hypothesis | |
|---|---|---|
| **Decision from the Clinical Trial** | Actually True | Actually wrong |
| **Null Hypothesis is true** | Right decision | Type II error |
| **Null Hypothesis is false** | Type I error | Right Decision |

Type I error is also called level significance and denoted by $\alpha$.

Type II error is denoted by $\beta$ and **(1- $\beta$)** is known as power of the test

Readers are encouraged to refer to the author's book for more details

Essentials of Bio-Statistics: An overview with the help of Software

ISBN: 978-1723712074

## Sample size determination

Sample size determination is one of the important tasks in the clinical trials as it ensures the statistical tests used in the analysis stage have sufficient power and validity. The general formula for calculating sample size includes the following parameters: Power of the test, Level of significance, Effect size and other parameters such as population rate & dropout rate.

The actual sample size calculation differs with respect to the nature of the outcome variable and the nature of the hypothesis (i.e. outcome variable is discrete or continuous variable and also whether the outcome variable is a numeric quantity or proportion). The following sections will discuss various types of sample size calculation using software.

## Effect size

Effect size is the difference between the treatment group and control group in terms of the main outcome variable. Here in our lung cancer example above, the main outcome variable is survival rate. The absolute effect size in this case is calculated as

Effect size = Treatment group survival rate – Control Group Survival rate

## Cohen Standard effect size

But Cohen defined the standard effect size in terms of small, medium and large for different measures.

## Cohen d effect size

Cohen's d effect size in case of comparison of survival time between standard drug and new drug group is calculated as follows:

$$\text{Cohen d} = \frac{Mean1 - Mean2}{\sqrt{(\sigma1\text{^}2) + (\sigma2\text{^}2)}}$$

Where

Mean1 = Mean survival time of new drug group

Mean2 = Mean survival time of new standard drug group

$\sigma1$ = standard deviation of survival time of the new drug group

$\sigma2$ = standard deviation of survival time of the standard drug group

Mean is a measure of central tendency and here mean survival time is central value of the variable survival time. Standard deviation is the square of variance which is a measure of deviation of values from its mean i.e. from mean survival time.

**R software package for Sample size determination**

We will be using the R statistical open source package to carry out the example of sample size calculations. Several packages which are developed by R community help the user to save time and efforts. The R software can be downloaded from the following link: **https://cran.r-project.org/**.

To make the working environment easier we can use R Studio which is a Graphical User Interface for the R Software. R Studio can be downloaded from the following link **https://www.rstudio.com/**.

The following r packages are used generally for the sample size calculations

1.      pwr package
2.      SampleSize4ClinicalTrials
3.      samplesize package
4.      TOSTER package
5.      PowerUpR package

We will be using pwr to calculate the sample size

### i. Sample size calculation for difference between proportions

Let us take an example of testing the difference in survival rate between two groups i.e. standard and new drug group. Let us define the following parameters for sample size calculations

Null Hypothesis Ho: Survival rate of new drug (s1) = Survival rate of standard drug (s2)

Null Hypothesis H1: Survival rate of new drug (s1) is greater than Survival rate of standard drug(s2)

Level of significance = 0.05

Power of the test = 0.8

Let s1= 0.3 and s2 = 0.25

The following codes needs to be feed into left most window of the R Studio environment

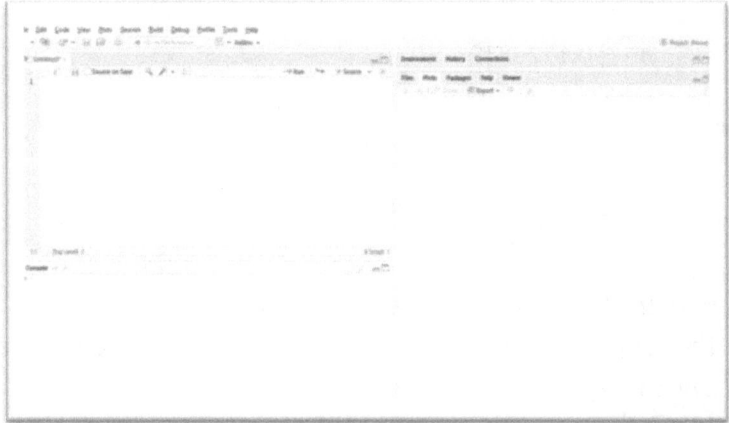

The pwr package needs to installed

**Installing the required packages**

**Install.packages(pwr)**

The package needs to be called into R studio environment

**Defining the pwr package in the R studio environment**
**Library(pwr)**

Compute the effect size using ES function and Cohen's standard effect size using cohen.ES

**Cohen Standard effect size calculation**

Let us consider s1= 0.3 and s2 = 0.25
**ES1 <- ES.h(p1= 0.3, p2 = 0.25)**
**ES2 <- cohen.ES(test = "p", size = "small")**

The value of effect size and Cohen's standard effect is obtained as

| Output – Effect Size |
| --- |
| **ES1**<br>[1] 0.1120819<br>**ES2**<br>test = p<br>size = small<br>effect size = 0.2 |

Here the Cohen's standard effect size is obtained as 0.2
The sample size is calculated using the p.test function of the pwr package

**Sample size determination using p.test function**

**With normal effect size ES1**
SSC <- pwr.p.test(h=ES1, sig.level = 0.05,power = 0.8, alternative = "greater")
**With Cohen standard effect size**
SSC <- pwr.p.test(h=ES2, sig.level = 0.05,power = 0.8, alternative = "greater")

The calculated sample size with standard effect size is obtained as follows

| Output – Sample size |
| --- |
| **With Normal Effect size** |
| proportion power calculation for binomial distribution (arcsine transformation)<br><br>h = 0.1120819<br>n = 492.1494<br>sig.level = 0.05<br>power = 0.8<br>alternative = greater |

From the above table we can get the required sample size for the clinical trial will be 492 which will be the sample size for each group

The power vs sample size curve can be obtained using

| Plotting power vs sample size |
| --- |
| plot(SSC) |

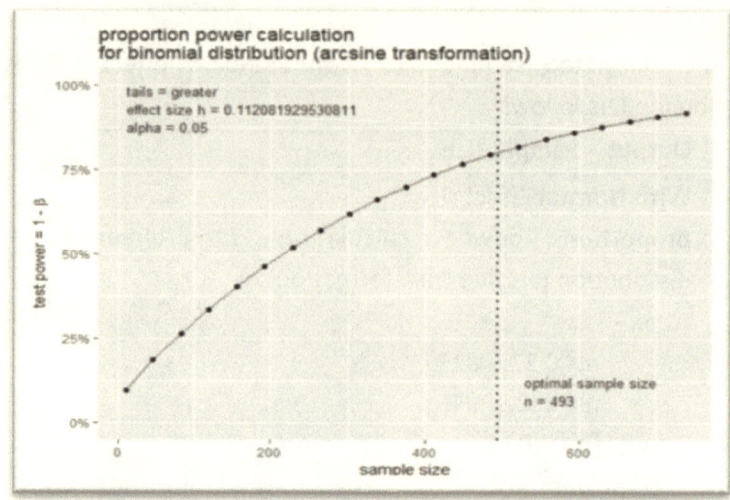

The calculated sample size with Cohen standard effect size is obtained as follows

| Output – Sample size |
| --- |
| **With Cohen standard  Effect size** |
| proportion power calculation for binomial distribution (arcsine transformation) |
| h = 0.2 |
| n = 154.5639 |
| sig.level = 0.05 |
| power = 0.8 |
| alternative = greater |

From the above table we can get the required sample size for the clinical trial will be 154 which will be the sample size for each group

The power vs sample size curve can be obtained using

| Plotting power vs sample size |
| --- |
| plot(SSC) |

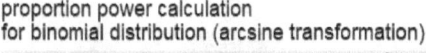

proportion power calculation
for binomial distribution (arcsine transformation)

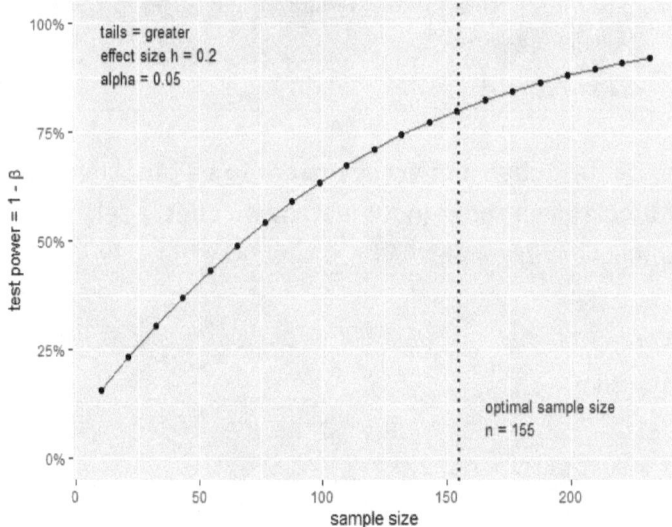

## Sample size calculation for difference between means

Let us take an example of testing the difference in mean survival time (in days) between two groups i.e. standard and new drug group. Let us define the following parameters for sample size calculations

Null Hypothesis Ho: Mean Survival time of new drug (m1) = Mean time of standard drug (m2)

Null Hypothesis H1: Mean Survival time of new drug (m1) is greater than Mean Survival time of standard drug (m2)

Level of significance = 0.05

Power of the test = 0.8

Let m1= 1485, m2 = 1465, s1 = 50 and s2 = 55

The mean and Standard deviation values needs to be taken from the previous studies or based on the population characteristics if it is known for estimating the sample size

The power package needs to be called into R studio environment

| Defining the pwr package in the R studio environment |
|---|
| Library(pwr) |

Compute the Cohen d effect size needs to be calculated from the formula given above (not the standard effect size)

| Cohen d calculation |
|---|
| M1<-1485 |
| M2<-1465 |
| sd1<-50 |
| sd2<-55 |
| sdc<-sqrt(sd1^2+sd2^2) |
| cohend<-(M1-M2)/sdc |

| Output – Cohen d Effect Size |
|---|
| cohend |
| [1] 0.2690691 |

Here the Cohen d effect size is 0.26

The sample size is calculated using the t.test function of the pwr package

| Sample size determination using t.test function |
|---|
| t1-<pwr.t.test(d=cohend, sig.level=.05, power = .80,alternative="greater" ) |

The sample size is obtained as

## Output – Sample size

Two-sample t test power calculation

n = 171.4736
d = 0.2690691
sig.level = 0.05
power = 0.8
alternative = greater
NOTE: n is number in *each* group

From the above table we can get the required sample size for the clinical trial will be 171 for each group
The power vs sample size curve can be obtained using

## Plotting power vs sample size

plot(t1)

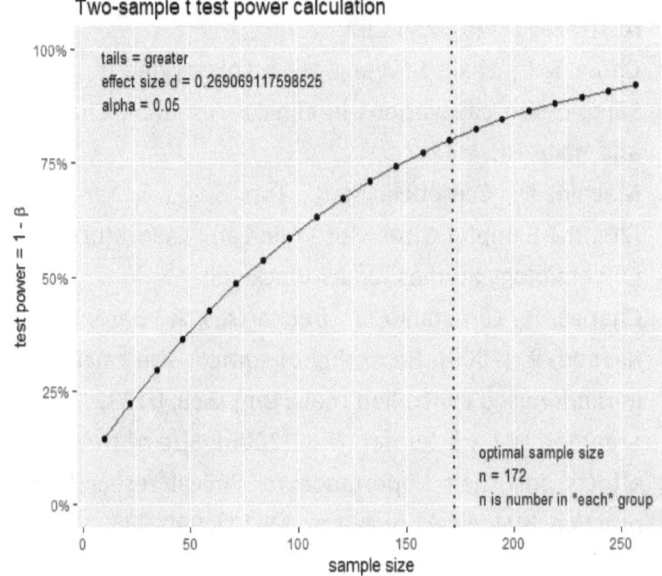

**References**

1. https://cran.r-project.org/web/packages/pwr/vignettes/pwr-vignette.html
2. https://cran.r-project.org/package=SampleSize4ClinicalTrials
3. https://cran.r-project.org/package=samplesize
4. https://cran.r-project.org/package=TOSTER
5. https://cran.r-project.org/package=PowerUpR
6. Cohen, J. (1988). Statistical power analysis for the behavioral sciences. Routledge.

7. Schoenfeld, D. A. (1983). Sample-size formula for the proportional-hazards regression model. Biometrics, 39(2), 499-503.
8. Kirby, A., Gebski, V., & Keech, A. C. (2002). Determining the sample size in a clinical trial. Medical journal of Australia, 177(5), 256-257.
9. Chow, S. C., Shao, J., Wang, H., & Lokhnygina, Y. (2017). Sample size calculations in clinical research. Chapman and Hall/CRC.
10. Machin, D., Campbell, M. J., Tan, S. B., & Tan, S. H. (2018). Sample Sizes for Clinical, Laboratory and Epidemiology Studies. Wiley-Blackwell.
11. Charles, P., Giraudeau, B., Dechartres, A., Baron, G., & Ravaud, P. (2009). Reporting of sample size calculation in randomised controlled trials. Bmj, 338, b1732.
12. Kraemer, H. C., & Kupfer, D. J. (2006). Size of treatment effects and their importance to clinical research and practice. Biological psychiatry, 59(11), 990-996.

13. Leon, A. C. (2008). Implications of clinical trial design on sample size requirements. Schizophrenia bulletin, 34(4), 664-669.

14. Dupont, W. D., & Plummer Jr, W. D. (1998). Power and sample size calculations for studies involving linear regression. Controlled clinical trials, 19(6), 589-601.

15. Perdices, M. (2018). Null hypothesis significance testing, p-values, effects sizes and confidence intervals. Brain Impairment, 19(1), 70-80.

16. Peace, K. E., & Chen, D. G. D. (2010). Clinical trial data analysis using R. CRC Press.

17. Grissom, R. J., & Kim, J. J. (2005). Effect sizes for research. A broad practical approach. Mah.

18. Sathian, B., Sreedharan, J., Baboo, S. N., Sharan, K., Abhilash, E. S., & Rajesh, E. (2010). Relevance of sample size determination in medical research. Nepal Journal of Epidemiology, 1(1), 4-10.

# Chapter 7 – Patient allocation and blinding

Randomization is an important part of the clinical trial process which helps us to arrive at valid results and free from allocation bias. Randomization ensures that the patients have equal chance of being assigned to different groups in the trial.

**Randomization Procedures**
There are different types of randomization procedures are available such as Simple randomization, Permuted block randomization, Stratified randomization and Adaptive randomization.

**Simple Randomization**
Simple randomization procedure involves assigning the patients into different treatment groups using a random number generator or flipping a coin. For example, the following are randomization sequence generated for two treatment groups 1 and 2 using the simple randomization procedure.
12112111112122211122
The simple randomization procedure is the simplest of all the randomization procedure but the main drawback of the simple randomization procedure is that the generated random allocation might be imbalance i.e. it will not ensure that the same number of patients is allocated to the two groups. Here the first group was allocated 12 and the second group was allocated only 8 patients.

**Permuted Block Randomization**

Permuted Block Randomization overcomes the problem of unequal sample size allocation. The overall sample size is divided into number of blocks with equal or unequal size.

For example our total sample size is 30 and we have to allocate 15 patients to each group. Here we can consider 5 blocks of size 6 with each block contains exactly 3 patients per group.

Each blocks of size 6 with two treatments can generate $^6C_2 =$ 15 combination of treatment blocks with 3 per each treatment as follows:

1.  121212
2.  212121
3.  111222
4.  222111
5.  112212
6.  221121
7.  122211
8.  211122
9.  112221
10. 221112
11. 122112
12. 211221
13. 112122
14. 221211
15. 122121

Now we have to select 5 blocks from the above 15 blocks using random number generator having number between 1 and 15. For example if the selected block numbers are 12, 3, 6,12,4 then the selected random sequence would be

211221111222221121211221222111

From the above allocation we can observe that the same number of patients are allocated in each group i.e. 15 patients per group at the end while ensuring the random allocation.

The drawback of this method of randomization is if the investigator came to know that 3 patients are allocated to a treatment group in a block then he can predict that the remaining patients will be allocated to other group only. To avoid this we can use blocks of different size.

### Stratified Randomization

Stratified randomization helps us to make the groups equal in terms of the independent or prognostic variables such as age, gender and severity of the disease condition. For example, the total sample is first divided by variable gender i.e. male and female patients and then under each category patients are allocated to different treatment groups by simple or permuted block randomization.

### Adaptive Randomization

Adaptive randomization procedure takes into account the prior allocation and adjusts the probability of allocating future patients to overcome the imbalance problem. There are different types of adaptive randomization procedures available such as urn randomization, biased coin randomization and another is minimization method.

In urn randomization procedure if there are two treatment groups are there then the each patient group is assigned a label or ball and when a particular balls is selected then the corresponding patient will be allocated to that group.

Here if the selected patient is from the first treatment group then one more ball from the second group will be added to the urn to reduce the imbalance or increase the probability of selecting the patient from the second treatment group.

In biased coin randomization method, if a group is allocated lesser number of patients then the next patients will have higher probability of being assigned to that group and vice versa.

In minimization method, imbalance score is calculated for each independent or prognostic variable and the patients will be allocated based on the randomization which minimizes the imbalance score with respect to different sub categories based on the prognostic variables. This procedure controls the imbalance at the prognostic variable level also.

**R code for simple randomization procedure**

| Simple randomization procedure |
| --- |
| #We need to install the randomizeR package |
| Install.package(randomizeR) |
| #Define the package in R environment |
| library(randomizeR) |
| #use crPar and genSeq function to generate random sequence of 2 groups from the sample size of 10 |
| random1 <- crPar(10,2) |
| randomsequence <- genSeq(random1) |

| Output |
| --- |
| Object of class "crPar" |
| design = CR |
| N = 10 |
| groups = A B |

```
[,1] [,2] [,3] [,4] [,5] [,6] [,7] [,8] [,9] [,10]
[1,] "A" "A" "A" "A" "A" "B" "B" "A" "A" "B"
```

The above code generated the simple randomization sequence for sample size of 10 with two treatment groups with 7 patients in group A and 3 Patients group B.

**R code for block randomization procedure**

| Block randomization procedure |
|---|
| #We need to install the randomizeR package |
| Install.package(psych) |
| #Define the package in R environment |
| library(psych) |
| #create block randomization with 5 block of size 2 with 1 for each treatment |
| random2 <- block.random(n=10,2) |
| random2 |

| Output | | |
|---|---|---|
| | blocks | IV1 |
| S1 | 1 | 1 |
| S2 | 1 | 2 |
| S3 | 2 | 2 |
| S4 | 2 | 1 |
| S5 | 3 | 2 |
| S6 | 3 | 1 |
| S7 | 4 | 1 |
| S8 | 4 | 2 |
| S9 | 5 | 2 |
| S10 | 5 | 1 |

Here block randomization ensured that the two treatments have same number of patients allocated.

## R code for block and stratified randomization procedure

**Stratified and Block randomization procedure**

```
#Define the package in R environment
library(psych)
#create block randomization with 5 block of size 2 with 1
for each treatment
random3 <- block.random(n=18,c(gender=2,disease=3))
random3
```

**Output**

| | blocks | gender | disease | treat |
|-----|--------|--------|---------|-------|
| S1 | 1 | 1 | 1 | 2 |
| S2 | 1 | 2 | 1 | 2 |
| S3 | 1 | 2 | 3 | 2 |
| S4 | 1 | 1 | 3 | 1 |
| S5 | 1 | 2 | 2 | 2 |
| S6 | 1 | 1 | 2 | 2 |
| S7 | 1 | 1 | 2 | 1 |
| S8 | 1 | 1 | 1 | 1 |
| S9 | 1 | 2 | 1 | 1 |
| S10 | 1 | 2 | 2 | 1 |
| S11 | 1 | 2 | 3 | 1 |
| S12 | 1 | 1 | 3 | 2 |
| S13 | 2 | 1 | 2 | 1 |
| S14 | 2 | 1 | 1 | 1 |
| S15 | 2 | 2 | 3 | 2 |
| S16 | 2 | 2 | 2 | 2 |
| S17 | 2 | 2 | 3 | 1 |
| S18 | 2 | 1 | 1 | 2 |
| S19 | 2 | 2 | 1 | 2 |
| S20 | 2 | 1 | 2 | 2 |
| S21 | 2 | 1 | 3 | 1 |
| S22 | 2 | 1 | 3 | 2 |
| S23 | 2 | 2 | 1 | 1 |
| S24 | 2 | 2 | 2 | 1 |

Here the two treatment groups are allocated randomly using 2 blocks and 2 factors gender (2 levels) and disease condition (3 levels).

**Stratified and Block randomization procedure**

```
#create stratified and block randomization plot using
panels function
pairs.panels(random3)
```

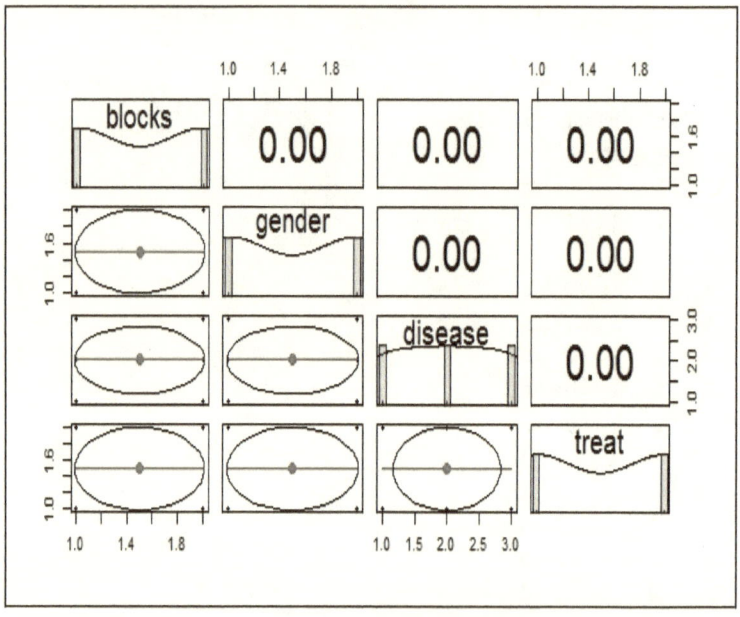

**R code for biased coin randomization procedure**

Biased coin randomization procedure

```
#Define the package in R environment
library(randomizeR)
#create Generalized Biased coin allocation with rho>0
myPar <- gbcdPar(10, 2)
genSeq(myPar)
```

```
Output
design = gbcd(2)
seed = 830081482
N = 10
groups = A B
rho = 2
The sequence M:

1 B A B A B A A B A B
```

The above output shows that the treatment allocation is balanced between groups.

## Blinding in Clinical Trials

Blinding in clinical trials helps us to reduce the bias in allocation of treatment and obtain valid results. The participant, the investigator and the analyst also can be blinded from the treatment allocation. Normally clinical trials are double blinded i.e. participants and the investigator.

## Inclusion and exclusion criteria

Clinical trials should define the inclusion criteria for selecting the patients into clinical trial and the criteria may be defined in terms of age, gender and prognosis factors and exclusion criteria may be defined as excluding pregnant women, patients with certain disease conditions and patients less than certain age due to risk involved in the clinical trial. It will be determined before the randomization process.

## Informed consent

Informed consent is an integral part of any clinical trial which needs to be obtained from patients towards meeting the legal and ethical requirements. The informed consent should be obtained from the participants before the start of the trial.

The informed consent is a tool which helps the participant to take decision to participate or not to participate in a clinical study. The informed consent form should contain important information related to the study and also should be in a language which the participant understands.

The informed consent needs to contain the following information about the trial

1.      Statement on aim and purpose of the clinical trial
2.      Potential benefits and risk involved in the trial
3.      Confidentiality of information
4.      Contact information related to the agency and investigators

5.  Statement about the voluntary participation in the trial
6.  Statement on possible injuries during the trial
7.  Statement on voluntary withdrawal during the trial
8.  Signature of the participant

In the case of children involved in the trial, consent must also be obtained from Parents and authorized representatives (apart from obtaining assent from Children if possible).

**Reference**

1. Kent, W. (2012). Randomisation and blinding in clinical trials.
2. Revelle, W., & Revelle, M. W. (2015). Package 'psych'. The Comprehensive R Archive Network.
3. Uschner, D., Schindler, D., Hilgers, R. D., & Heussen, N. (2018). randomizeR: an R package for the assessment and implementation of randomization in clinical trials. Journal of Statistical Software, 85(8), 1-22.
4. **https://cran.r-project.org/web/packages/psych/index.html**
5. **https://cran.r-project.org/package=randomizeR**
6. Nguyen, T. L., Collins, G. S., Lamy, A., Devereaux, P. J., Daurès, J. P., Landais, P., & Le Manach, Y. (2017). Simple randomization did not protect against bias in smaller trials. Journal of clinical epidemiology, 84, 105-113.
7. Broglio, K. (2018). Randomization in clinical trials: permuted blocks and stratification. Jama, 319(21), 2223-2224.
8. Wathen, J. K., & Thall, P. F. (2017). A simulation study of outcome adaptive randomization in multi-arm clinical trials. Clinical Trials, 14(5), 432-440.
9. Speich, B. (2017). Blinding in surgical randomized clinical trials in 2015. Annals of surgery, 266(1), 21-22.

# Chapter 8 – Data collection and Data monitoring during the clinical trial

**Case Report Forms (CRFs) or e-Case Report Forms (e-CRF)**

After the preparation of clinical trial protocol, the next step involved in the clinical trial process is to collect the data from the participants. Usually the data collection and recording instrument in the clinical trial is referred as Case Report Form (CRF) or nowadays called e-CRF as the data is collected electronically. Standardized CRFs enable the investigator or sponsor of the clinical trials to carry out effective and efficient data analysis and helps them to prepare the final trial reports.

Food and Drug Administration (FDA) organization of United States of America introduced 21 CRF Part II regulations for acceptance of electronic records and electronic signature instead of paper forms.

Medical coding during the clinical trials is carried out using standard dictionaries such as Medical Dictionary for Regulatory Activities (MedDRA) and World Health Organisation Drug Dictio-nary Enhanced (WHO-DDE).

CRFs in the form of multiple forms contains the following information such as (not limited to)

1. Patient demographic details
2. Inclusion and exclusion criteria
3. Randomization details
4. Informed consent details
5. Medical history
6. Physical examination measurement,

7.   Vital signs measurements
8.   Laboratory measurements
9.   Visit details
10.  Prior and concomitant medication details
11.  Drug/treatment administration details with time line,
     12.  Adverse event log.
     13.  Other Information per protocol
     14.  Evaluation of medication/treatment response

**Validation of and audit of data collected through e-CRFs**

The validation of data collected through e-CRFs can be achieved by including the validation at the data entry level to prevent any missing data, correct range of values for a particular data field, ensuring correct data format. Data quality audit to be carried out to ensure the data is collected as per the clinical trial protocol. Database will be locked after all the data collection process is completed in a trial to avoid any manipulation during the final analysis stage.

**Clinical Data interchange Standards Consortium**

Clinical Data Interchange Standards Consortium (CDISC) is a non-governmental organization which develops platform independent data standards to enable interoperability of information generated during the clinical trials and clinical research. The standard has two parts one is foundational standards and another is data exchange standards.

**Foundational standards include**
   i.    Protocol,
   ii.   Study design,
   iii.  Clinical Data Acquisition Standards Harmonization (CDASH),
   iv.   Laboratory Data Model (LAB),

v. Study Data Tabulation Model (SDTM)
vi. Standard Exchange of Non-Clinical Data (SEND)
vii. Analysis Data Model (ADaM)

**Data Exchange standards**
i. Study/ Trial Design Model - eXtensible Markup Language (SDM-XML)
ii. Operational Data Model
iii. Define eXtensible Markup Language (XML)

Both the standards cover the data collection and data exchange aspect of the clinical trials.

Current data collection process in the clinical trials integrates the electronic health records, wearable devices, mobile applications, cloud computing storage,

Readers can refer author's book on "Application of statistical tools in biomedical domain: An overview with help of software" for further information about the clinical trial data management.

**https://www.amazon.com/dp/B07BWRCW5F.**

**Clinical Trial Data Monitoring Committee**

Data monitoring committee role in clinical trials is to review the data collection process, adherence to the clinical trial protocol, assess the efficacy and safety of the treatments. The role includes reporting of adverse events, ethical and safety issues arising during the conduct of clinical trial. Based on the review the committee may recommend the stopping of the clinical trial or withdrawal of participants due to safety issues.

**Reference**

1. Bellary, S., Krishnankutty, B., & Latha, M. S. (2014). Basics of case report form designing in clinical research. Perspectives in clinical research, 5(4), 159.

2.  Le Jeannic, A., Quelen, C., Alberti, C., & Durand-Zaleski, I. (2014). Comparison of two data collection processes in clinical studies: electronic and paper case report forms. BMC medical research methodology, 14(1), 7.

3.  Ellenberg, S. S., Fleming, T. R., & DeMets, D. L. (2019). Data monitoring in clinical trials: a practical perspective. STATISTICS IN PRACTICE.

4.  Hume, S. (2017). CLINICAL DATA MANAGEMENT. Applied Clinical Trials, 25(2/3), 19.

5.  **https://www.cdisc.org/**

# Chapter 9 – Statistical Analysis in clinical trial

Statistical Analysis Plan (SAP) is prepared before the start of the trial which forms the basis of analyzing the data during the clinical trial. It contains the following components:

1.     Defines of the hypothesis
2.     Population under study
3.     Parameters, variables and covariates
4.     Primary and surrogate endpoints
5.     Sample size considerations
6.     statistical tools and tests
7.     Interim Analysis plan
8.     Intention to Treat analysis (ITT)
9.     Subgroup analysis
10.    Statistical software packages used in trial
11.    Timing of analysis
12.    Safety monitoring analysis
13.    Missing data management

**Primary and Surrogate endpoints**
Primary endpoint is the outcome of the clinical trial and when the primary endpoint is not measurable surrogate end point will be used which is a close but not exactly the same as the primary endpoint.

**Interim Analysis plan**
Interim analysis plan is an important tool which helps us to ensure that the trial is safe and can be continued. It defines the stopping rules based on the safety issues or evidence of highly beneficial treatment is seen.

## Intention to treat analysis

Intention to treat analysis includes the analytical methods which takes into account the original randomization schedule even when the patient violated the trial protocol and did not receive the actual treatment which was assigned to the patient.

## Sub group analysis

Sub group analysis is carried out on primary end point with respect to subgroups defined based on baseline characteristics such as gender and age of the participants.

## Statistical tools and tests used in the clinical trial

Different types of statistical tools and tests will be used based on the trial objective, design and protocol. Following are the commonly used statistical tools and tests in clinical trial. Readers are encouraged to refer to the author's book on "Essentials of Bio-Statistics: An overview with the help of Software" **https://www.amazon.com/dp/B07GRBXX7D**.

1. Descriptive statistics
a. Mean
b. Variance and Standard deviations
2. Correlation and regression
3. Estimation and confidence interval
a. Confidence interval for proportion
b. Confidence interval for mean
4. Hypothesis testing
a. Testing single Proportion
b. Testing single Mean
c. Difference in proportion
d. Difference in mean
5. Analysis of Variance(ANOVA)
6. Repeated Measures ANOVA

7. Sensitivity, specificity, odds ratio, relative risk. ROC curve analysis
8. Principal Component analysis
9. Survival Analysis

**Statistical software packages**
There are number of statistical software packages used in the clinical trials
1.    Statistical Analysis System (SAS)
2.    STATA
3.    Statistical Packages of Social Science(SPSS IBM)
4.    R

**Reference**
1. Gamble, C., Krishan, A., Stocken, D., Lewis, S., Juszczak, E., Doré, C., ... & Berlin, J. (2017). Guidelines for the content of statistical analysis plans in clinical trials. Jama, 318(23), 2337-2343.
2. Yuan, I., Topjian, A. A., Kurth, C. D., Kirschen, M. P., Ward, C. G., Zhang, B., & Mensinger, J. L. (2019). Guide to the statistical analysis plan. Pediatric Anesthesia, 29(3), 237-242.
3. McCoy C. E. (2017). Understanding the Intention-to-treat Principle in Randomized Controlled Trials. The western journal of emergency medicine, 18(6), 1075–1078. doi:10.5811/westjem.2017.8.35985
4. Kumar, A., & Chakraborty, B. S. (2016). Interim analysis: A rational approach of decision making in clinical trial. Journal of advanced pharmaceutical technology & research, 7(4), 118.

5. Delgado-Herrera, L., & Anbar, D. (2003). A model for the interim analysis process:: a case study. Controlled clinical trials, 24(1), 51-65.

6. Dembe, A. E., Partridge, J. S., & Geist, L. C. (2011). Statistical software applications used in health services research: analysis of published studies in the US. BMC health services research, 11(1), 252.

7. Prajapati, K., Kumar, P., & Solutions, G. C. E. Exploring Use of R for Clinical Trials.

8. **https://www.r-project.org/doc/R-FDA.pdf**

9. Wang, R., Lagakos, S. W., Ware, J. H., Hunter, D. J., & Drazen, J. M. (2007). Statistics in medicine—reporting of subgroup analyses in clinical trials. New England Journal of Medicine, 357(21), 2189-2194.

10. Ballarini, N., Chiu, Y. D., König, F., Posch, M., & Jaki, T. (2018). Graphical displays for subgroup analysis in clinical trials.

11. Hollis, S., & Campbell, F. (1999). What is meant by intention to treat analysis? Survey of published randomised controlled trials. Bmj, 319(7211), 670-674.

12. Kruse, R. L., Alper, B. S., Reust, C., Stevermer, J. J., Shannon, S., & Williams, R. H. (2002). Intention-to-treat analysis: Who is in? Who is out?. Journal of Family Practice, 51(11), 969-971.

13. Pocock, S. J. (1982). Interim analyses for randomized clinical trials: the group sequential approach. Biometrics, 153-162.

# Chapter 10 – Reporting in clinical trial

Regulatory authorities like Food and Drug Administration (FDA) organization requires the clinical trials results are reported as per the standards lay down by them. Reporting of Clinical Trials is mandatory in the United States of America

The following details to be provided for the registration of clinical trials

1. Information about the trial
a. Title
b. Aim and summary
c. Study design
d. Phase of clinical trial
e. Type of clinical trial
f. Primary disease or condition studied in the trial
g. Treatments being used
h. Start and end date of the study
i. Primary and secondary outcome measures
2. Participant selection and recruitment information
3. Contact information

The following are components to be present in the final result report which will be submitted for FDA approval:

1. Participant flow
2. Demographic and Baseline characteristics
3. Outcomes measures and statistical analysis
4. Adverse event
5. Protocol and Statistical Analysis Plan (SAP)
6. Trial sponsor information

www.ingramcontent.com/pod-product-compliance
Lightning Source LLC
Chambersburg PA
CBHW030735180526
45157CB00008BA/3175